The Habit Shift

A Lifestyle Approach to Sustainable Weight Loss

Dr. Melissa Ramsey
DNP, MSN, RN, FNP-C

Table of Contents

My Story

I became aware of my size at a very young age—around twelve. I remember sitting in the doctor's office when he told me I needed to lose weight. In that moment, embarrassment washed over me. I didn't fully understand what that meant, but I knew it wasn't good. I wondered what was wrong with me. Why did I have to deal with something that none of my friends seemed to struggle with?

At family gatherings, I can still recall the comments that were meant to be helpful but cut deep instead. "You have such a pretty face." "You'd be so cute if you just lost a little weight." I know now that my family meant well, but at the time, those words made me feel small and exposed. Their concern, though rooted in love, made me self-conscious and ashamed of my body. Eventually, I started to cope the only way I knew how— by turning to food for comfort. It was the one thing that never judged me. But the more I ate to feel better, the more weight I gained.

Sometimes, I just avoided the situation altogether. I'd skip family events to avoid hearing the comments or seeing the looks that made me feel like I was disappointing someone. Deep down, I just wanted this problem to disappear. I wanted to feel normal, but I had no idea where to turn or how to make that happen.

To make matters worse, finding clothes that fit was almost impossible. My mom ended up sewing most of my outfits because, growing up in the late '80s and early '90s, clothing for curvier girls didn't exist. This was long before J. Lo and Beyoncé made curves something to be celebrated. Back then, they were something to be hidden. I remember feeling so out of place, showing up to school in dresses that looked more suited for church or an office than for a teenager. I would stand in front of the mirror, tugging at my clothes, wishing I could just blend in.

At night, I would pray and ask God, "Why me? Why can't I just be a normal size like the other girls?" I didn't want to stand out; I just wanted to fit in.

Then, during high school, I had a close friend who was also overweight. At the start of one school year, she lost about twenty pounds. I was so happy for her—and secretly a little jealous. I wanted that same transformation for myself. I remember asking her what she did, and she told me she started exercising and eating less. That was all the information I got. We were only fifteen or sixteen—what did we really know about calories, fat, or nutrition? Still, those few words stuck with me. Somewhere inside, a spark was lit. I thought, *maybe I can do that too.*

The Habit Shift

I started eating what I thought "people on diets" were supposed to eat. I would eat very small portions and exercise every day. The weight came off, but I was constantly hungry. I'd lose a few pounds, then eventually give in—either because of hunger or being around other people's food. Looking back, I believe that's when my struggles with binge eating began, though I didn't recognize it at the time. All I knew was that if I ate less, the scale would go down.

During my senior year of high school, I started paying closer attention to what I ate. I tried to include more protein and slightly larger portions, but I still kept things very controlled. I set rigid eating schedules and time frames, all with the goal of looking a certain way by graduation. Even when I was hungry, I would remind myself of that goal and push through.

Around this time, I decided to start running—just like my mom. My mom used to run for what felt like hours. I could never quite understand why she enjoyed running in circles, but what I did know was that she looked amazing. She could always fit into her clothes, eat what she wanted, and still maintain her weight. I wanted that for myself.

So, I started small—running laps around our backyard pool. It wasn't exactly the most practical setup, but it felt like a safe place to start. I was shy and didn't want anyone to see me exercising. The thought of running around the neighborhood where my friends might see me was mortifying. I wanted to change, but I didn't want to draw attention to myself while doing it. Eventually, my backyard running days ended when I was told to stop because I was ruining the grass!

That's when I had no choice but to go to the track. The first time I ran there, I realized just how small my "laps" around the pool really were—it was both humbling and funny. But being at the track gave me something new: a way to measure my progress. I could see how far I was going and how much I was improving, one lap at a time.

I started out slow, struggling to make it through even a single lap without stopping. But I kept showing up. One lap turned into two, then three, then four. Before I knew it, I was running five miles a day. By the time I graduated high school, I had gone from 230 pounds to 170 pounds.

That experience did more than change my body—it changed the way I saw myself. Running taught me discipline, consistency, and the power of setting a goal and sticking to it. It ignited my love for running, but even more importantly, it gave me confidence. I proved to myself that I could do hard things—and no one could take that feeling away.

College Years & Weight Struggle

When I started college, I was full of excitement and ready to begin my new chapter. I had been accepted to Tuskegee University—miles away from home—and I was determined to make the most of it. I arrived with all the optimism and structure that had carried me through high school. I told myself I would keep running, eat sensibly, and stay in control of my weight.

But college life had other plans. The food was different, my schedule was packed, and the Southern heat was no joke. I had never experienced waking up to 90-degree weather before—it was suffocating. My morning runs quickly turned into quick excuses. I'd tell myself, I'll go tomorrow when it's cooler, but "tomorrow" rarely came. And truthfully, I was having fun—maybe for the first time in my life without constantly worrying about my body or the scale. For a little while, I wanted to be carefree like everyone else.

When I came home for the holidays, though, reality hit hard. I had regained some of the weight, and almost instantly, the comments started. Family members—once again meaning well—said things like, "Looks like the freshman twenty got you!" or "You must be enjoying that cafeteria food." What was supposed to be a happy, relaxing break turned into a source of shame. I felt like I had disappointed everyone, including myself.

Back at school, that shame followed me. I coped the only way I knew how—by trying to take control of my body again. But this time, I went to extremes. I started fasting and using laxatives, thinking I could undo the damage. I convinced myself it was discipline, but really, it was punishment.

My "fasting" was far from healthy. I would buy bottles of cranberry juice, fruit punch, and V8, then dilute them with water to make them last longer. I told myself it was enough to keep me going. The V8 was my trick—it was heavier, and I hoped it would keep my stomach from growling during class. The first few days were miserable, but after a while, the hunger pains faded. That was almost worse because I got used to it. I started to believe that ignoring hunger was strength.

By the time I came home for summer break, my family barely recognized me. I was down to around 140 pounds—the smallest I had ever been as an adult. To me, it felt like an accomplishment, but to them, it looked like something was wrong. Their concern was written all over their faces, and that made me more secretive. I learned to "perform" eating when I was around them—picking at food, pretending to be full—then going back to my diluted juice routine when I was alone. I had mastered the art of control, but it was control built on fear.

Adulthood and Realization

That cycle continued throughout my college years. When I finally graduated and returned home for good, I began to struggle again with my weight. But now, dieting has become an entire industry. There were always new trends promising quick results and permanent change. I told myself this one will be different every single time.

I tried them all—low-carb, intermittent fasting, even the cabbage soup diet. Each one started with hope and ended with disappointment. I would lose the weight quickly, feel proud for a short time, then gain it all back once I returned to eating normally. I even tried formal weight-loss programs, but I couldn't afford to stay on them long-term. So, I'd go to the grocery store and buy prepackaged meals, trying to recreate what I saw in the commercials. But no matter what I did, the outcome was the same.

It became a familiar pattern—lose the weight, gain it back, start over again. I was stuck in a loop, chasing a version of "success" that never seemed to last. And deep down, I was exhausted—not just physically, but emotionally. I wanted peace with my body, but I didn't yet know how to find it.

As time went on, I found different ways to keep my weight down, but no matter what method I used, the story always ended the same. I'd lose the weight, feel proud for a while, and then slowly, without even realizing it, the pounds would creep back on. Each time, I promised myself that this time would be different. But it never was.

Even during pregnancy, the cycle continued. Each time I became pregnant, I would gain at least 100 pounds. After giving birth, I would go right back to what I knew—running and eating less—and eventually lose the weight again. I became an expert at *losing* weight but never at *keeping* it off. My elusive goal wasn't just to be thin—it was to finally stay that way. I remember thinking, *How do people actually keep the weight off for good? What's their secret?*

I often heard people say, "You have to make it a lifestyle change." But honestly, I never understood what that really meant. To me, it sounded like they were saying I'd have to give up all the foods I loved forever. I didn't want a life without joy or flavor. I believed that once I reached my goal weight, I could simply go back to eating what I wanted, just in smaller portions. Time and time again, though, reality proved me wrong.

When I began my career as a registered nurse, I thought that having more knowledge about health would help me manage my weight better. But even then, the pattern stayed the same. I worked in the coronary care unit, and because I worked the night shift, I often had quiet moments to talk to my patients. Those late-night conversations changed me in ways I didn't realize at the time. Many of my patients were older adults recovering from heart attacks or heart surgery, and they often opened up about their regrets. Over and over, I heard the same words: *"If I could do life over again, I would have made healthier choices."*

Those words stayed with me. Here I was—a nurse, someone who taught others about wellness and disease prevention—listening to their stories while still fighting my own silent battle with food and weight. I was living proof that knowledge alone wasn't enough to create change.

Ironically, I *loved* exercise. I even became a group fitness instructor. Teaching classes gave me the confidence I'd never known before. The shy girl who used to avoid attention was now leading rooms full of people, music pumping, motivating others to move their bodies. It felt incredible. Exercise became my outlet, my escape, and my stage. But even with all that activity, I couldn't seem to conquer the part of the journey that mattered most—nutrition. I knew I was strong, capable, and fit, but "diet control" still felt like this distant, impossible dream.

The Elusive "Lifestyle Change"

Through my research, three key behaviors consistently stood out as powerful contributors to weight loss success. The first was drinking enough water—at least 80 ounces a day. Studies show that staying well-hydrated can prevent confusing thirst with hunger, which often leads to unnecessary snacking. When you drink enough water, your body functions more efficiently, digestion improves, and cravings tend to decrease.

The second finding was the importance of meal prepping and planning. This proved to be the single most influential factor in long-term weight loss success. When individuals knew what they were going to eat—and had it prepared ahead of time—they were far less likely to make impulsive or unhealthy food choices. Having a plan eliminates decision fatigue and helps you stay aligned with your goals, even on busy days.

Lastly, incorporating regular exercise—just 20 to 30 minutes of movement each day—made a significant difference. This doesn't have to mean intense workouts; even walking, stretching, or light strength training supports progress. Consistent movement not only helps the scale move in the right direction but also boosts mood, reduces stress, and improves overall health.

These three foundational habits—hydration, preparation, and movement—may seem simple, but when practiced consistently, they create the structure necessary for lasting success.

In 2020, the world seemed to turn upside down, and with it came new conversations about health—and new solutions. I started hearing about weight loss injections, medications that could help suppress appetite. I remember thinking, *Wow, that must be nice—to not feel hungry all the time and still lose weight.* I was curious, but at that point, I hadn't seriously considered trying them myself.

That same year, my sister and I decided to open a wellness center. It was exciting but also one of the most stressful times of my life. We started by offering B12 injections and weight loss medications to clients. I was helping others on their weight loss journeys while still quietly struggling with my own. And if starting a new business wasn't stressful enough, I also made the decision to go back to school to get my doctorate. Talk about pressure. Between running a business, studying, and trying to balance life, stress became my constant companion.

And history had already shown me how I responded to stress—I ate.

In 2020, I came across peptides just as they were beginning to gain popularity in the world of health and wellness. I was intrigued but also hesitant. After years of seeing new diets, detoxes, and "miracle" solutions come and go, part of me wondered if this was just another fad. Still, something about the science behind peptides caught my attention—it seemed more evidence-based, more physiological, and less gimmicky than what I had seen before.

Around that same time, I began my doctoral program, focusing on obesity and weight management. The timing felt almost serendipitous. I had lived this struggle personally for decades, and now I had the opportunity to study it from a scientific and behavioral standpoint. Through my coursework and early research, one consistent theme stood out across the literature: Cognitive Behavioral Therapy (CBT).

I knew early on that my dissertation would center around treatments for obesity, but I wasn't yet sure which direction it would take. As I delved deeper, I became fascinated by how often CBT appeared in the research—not just as a therapy for mental health, but as a powerful tool for sustainable weight management. CBT has long been used to treat anxiety and depression by helping individuals recognize and modify maladaptive behaviors (Fernández-Álvarez & Fernández-Álvarez, 2019). It's about retraining the mind—learning to identify the thoughts and emotions that drive our behaviors, and then consciously replacing old, unhelpful patterns with new, productive ones.

The more I read, the more it became clear that this same process could be transformative for people struggling with weight. The evidence was compelling. Studies showed that incorporating CBT principles into obesity treatment improved long-term outcomes and reduced relapse rates (Andrew et al., 2020; Angelidi et al., 2021; Bray et al., 2018; Campbell-Danesh, 2020; Chopra et al., 2021; Dalle Grave et al., 2020; Gadde & Atkins, 2020; Hall & Kahan, 2018, 2019). Unlike short-term diets or rigid exercise plans, CBT focuses on *why* people eat the way they do—and how their thoughts, emotions, and habits intertwine to either support or sabotage progress.

For the first time, I began to see obesity not as a personal failure or lack of discipline, but as a behavioral condition—something that could be approached through a structured, evidence-based framework. This realization shifted everything for me. It bridged the gap between what I had lived through personally and what I was now learning academically.

That research was a turning point for me—it revealed the missing piece in my lifelong struggle with weight: my mindset. For so long, I thought the problem was food. I believed that if I could just find the "right" diet, the "right" exercise routine, or the "right" motivation, I'd finally win the battle. But what I didn't realize was that my thoughts about food, my relationship with it, and the way I spoke to myself were quietly controlling everything.

Food was always on my mind. I could eat all day if I decided to, and sometimes, I did. I remember one of the lowest points in my life: I'd work night shifts, and when my husband and kids left for work and school in the morning, I would come home, exhausted, and instead of resting, I would raid the kitchen. I'd eat until I was painfully full—so full that standing up felt unbearable. I would sit there, ashamed, asking myself, *Why are you doing this? Why can't you stop?*

That cycle—restriction, binging, guilt, and self-punishment—was my normal for years. I had what I now recognize as an all-or-nothing mentality. If I slipped up, I was a failure. There was no middle ground. One cookie meant I'd already "ruined" the day, so I might as well eat whatever I wanted and start over on Monday. And when Monday came, I'd begin again—restricting myself, white-knuckling through hunger and cravings, only to binge again days later.

Looking back, I realize how hard I was on myself. I treated every slip-up like a moral failure instead of a human moment. I told myself things like, "You'll never get this right," or "You deserve to be overweight." My relationship with food was tangled up with shame, guilt, and punishment—and that mindset made lasting change impossible.

As I dove deeper into the research on Cognitive Behavioral Therapy, I began to see myself reflected in the patterns it described. CBT teaches that our thoughts shape our feelings, and our feelings drive our behaviors. My thoughts—*I failed again, I might as well eat, I'll start over later*—were fueling my behavior. I wasn't broken; I was simply caught in a destructive loop I didn't know how to interrupt.

I started to ask myself: *What if I could change that? What if I could retrain my thinking the same way I had trained my body to run five miles a day years ago?*

That question changed everything. I began experimenting with new ways of thinking. Instead of labeling food as "good" or "bad," I tried to see it as neutral—fuel that could either help or hinder my goals. When I overate, I practiced curiosity instead of criticism. I asked, *What was I feeling before I ate? Was I tired, lonely, stressed, or bored?* Slowly, I began to see that the key to long-term weight loss wasn't just discipline—it was self-awareness.

The truth is, most weight loss begins with a shift in mindset. The body simply follows what the mind believes. When I decided to eat well, I did. When I decided to indulge, I did that too. My body was only following my thoughts. I finally understood that I couldn't lose weight one way and expect to maintain it another. Whatever plan I followed had to be sustainable for life—not another temporary fix, but a new way of thinking, living, and being.

Obesity has become one of the most complex and widespread pandemics of our time, and without new strategies, the numbers will continue to rise. While many approaches focus on short-term solutions, lifestyle and behavioral changes address the deeper, psychological aspects of habits—and these often hold the key to lasting results. People pursue weight loss for different reasons: health, special events, or milestone moments. Yet, when the event passes, familiar patterns tend to return, and so does the weight.

Obesity is a chronic condition that can lead to serious health complications and even premature death if untreated. According to Khanna et al. (2022), individuals with a body mass index (BMI) of 30 or higher are considered obese. This is not a localized issue—it's a global one, with consequences that have continued to intensify. Adiposity affects people across all ages and in every region, from developing to developed nations. Among children ages 2 to 18, obesity rates—defined as a BMI greater than the 95th percentile—have climbed dramatically, from 54 percent in 2008 to 69 percent in 2017 (American Heart Association, 2018; Mayo Clinic, 2021; World Health Organization, 2020). These early patterns of obesity set the stage for chronic illnesses such as heart disease and diabetes later in life.

The global rise in obesity has been staggering. In 2008, an estimated 500 million adults—roughly 10 to 14 percent of the world's population—were considered obese. By 2016, that number had reached around 671 million. In the United States, adult obesity rates increased from 30.5 percent to 42.4 percent, and severe obesity nearly doubled, from 4.7 percent to 9.2 percent. The sharpest increases have been seen in Latin America, North America, North Africa, and the Middle East (Avnieli Velfer et al., 2019; Centers for Disease Control and Prevention, 2021; Chopra et al., 2020; Malik et al., 2020). I know the numbers may seem a bit daunting, but they add value and credibility to just how important this change truly is.

Many factors contribute to the development of obesity—excessive caloric intake, sedentary lifestyles, genetics, medications, and the pressures of modern living among them (Ansari & Elhag, 2021; Ansari et al., 2020; Mayle, 2021). Despite widespread awareness, rates continue to climb. For many, weight loss efforts last only a few months before old behaviors resurface. Studies have shown that attrition, or the loss of engagement in a weight loss program, is one of the most significant predictors of poor long-term outcomes (Ansari & Elhag, 2021; Dalle Grave et al., 2015; Everitt et al., 2022; Pirotta et al., 2019; Ponzo et al., 2020).

Habits are at the heart of this struggle. As Orvidas (2019) describes, a habit is formed when an incentive creates an impulse to act through learned stimulus-response patterns.

These habits can work for us—or against us. Cognitive Behavioral Therapy (CBT), widely recognized as the gold standard for treating anxiety and depression, focuses on transforming these maladaptive patterns into constructive, goal-oriented behaviors (Fernández-Álvarez & Fernández-Álvarez, 2019). CBT's success in mental health has led to its growing use in long-term obesity management, where behavior change is essential for sustainability (Andrew et al., 2020; Angelidi et al., 2021; Bray et al., 2018; Campbell-Danesh, 2020; Chopra et al., 2020; Chopra et al., 2021; Dalle Grave et al., 2020; Gadde & Atkins, 2020; Grave et al., 2020; Hall & Kahan, 2018, 2019; Iłowiecka et al., 2021; Krishnaswami et al., 2018; LeBlanc et al., 2018; Madjd et al., 2019; Moraes et al., 2021; Rand, 2017; Varkevisser et al., 2019).

Drawing upon these principles, I developed a 14-step program that merges CBT's core concepts with a practical, structured approach to weight loss. This program was built around common challenges people face when trying to lose weight, offering actionable strategies to overcome them sustainably. It provides a clear, evidence-based path for individuals to build healthier habits that last.

In my research, I combined the behavioral science of CBT with James Clear's framework for habit formation. This integration gave participants a simple and repeatable method to create lasting changes. Habit-tracking tools—whether physical calendars or digital apps—became a key part of the process, helping participants stay accountable, consistent, and mindful of their progress.

Fifty participants took part in the project, including five men and forty-five women. Each selected one habit to focus on for six weeks. The Self-Reported Habit Index (SRHI) was completed before and after the program to assess habit strength. Every participant who completed the SRHI showed improvement, with scores increasing by at least seven points. Within James Clear's Habit Tracker (JCHT), the top completion range was between 61 and 70 percent. Most participants who improved on the SRHI also maintained a JCHT completion rate of 50 percent or more. The data revealed a clear link—higher JCHT completion correlated with greater improvements in SRHI scores, suggesting that consistent tracking played a vital role in success.

The findings showed that the JCHT is not just a theoretical concept—it's a simple, effective tool that can be applied in community, inpatient, and outpatient settings. Once introduced by a healthcare provider, it empowers patients to take ownership of their progress and commit to sustainable change.

The 14 weekly focus points, combined with the habit tracker, serve as a long-term guide through this journey. They can be repeated whenever needed to strengthen habits or prevent relapse. It's best to start during a period free from major events—like vacations or celebrations—for at least 30 days, giving new habits time to take root.

When I began my own journey with peptides, I was determined not to fall into another cycle of quick fixes. I wanted this time to be different. I started by aligning CBT principles with the real-life obstacles my patients and I had faced. My goal was to create practical, compassionate solutions—ones rooted in self-awareness and sustainability rather than restriction or guilt. What I discovered was that true, lasting change isn't about perfection. It's about awareness, consistency, and kindness toward yourself.

Even while using peptides, I made balance my focus—learning how to nourish my body while still enjoying food. I used medication as a supportive tool, not a solution. I followed a structured meal plan and exercised regularly. Through this approach, I lost 80 pounds in ten months and, more importantly, have maintained that loss.

This is the longest I've ever stayed at my goal weight, and it's because I shifted my mindset. I stopped chasing a number and started building a lifestyle. When health becomes part of who you are—not something you're trying to reach—you no longer need to start over. My journey from 230 pounds to 160 pounds wasn't about restriction; it was about rediscovering balance and trust in myself.

The Habit Shift

Early on, I worked closely with a nutritionist who helped me develop a structured plan focused on high protein, moderate carbohydrates, and low fat. For years, I had struggled with what to eat and how much. This plan gave me clarity and freedom—it wasn't about dieting, but about nourishment. I began eating six balanced meals a day, each centered on protein, which helped me stay full, energized, and in control. Drinking plenty of water and moving regularly became second nature.

For the first time, I wasn't counting down the days of a "challenge." I was living differently. I allowed myself flexibility, including the occasional treat meal, without guilt. If I wanted pizza or dessert, I adjusted my meals for the day and enjoyed it. To my surprise, the scale didn't spike. That realization changed everything—it wasn't one indulgent day that derailed me before; it was the shame and "all-or-nothing" thinking that came after.

Learning to see food without guilt was one of the most freeing parts of this journey. I stopped labeling foods as good or bad and started seeing them as choices—each with its own consequence, but none deserving shame. This mindset, built through consistent habits and self-compassion, became the foundation of my lasting success.

In the end, I realized that sustainable weight loss isn't about willpower—it's about mindset. It's about creating systems that support your goals, practicing self-compassion, and showing up for yourself, even when progress feels slow. When I stopped punishing myself for past failures and started planning for future success, everything changed.

The Focus Points

The 14 focus points are the heart of this program. They are designed to address the most common setbacks I encountered on my weight loss journey while providing practical strategies to overcome them. Using the principles of cognitive behavioral therapy (CBT), these focus points gradually helped me retrain old patterns and replace them with habits that are sustainable over the long term.

This process requires time, patience, and consistency. The first time I implemented these strategies, I was far from perfect. I stumbled, made mistakes, and occasionally felt frustrated—but I learned to focus on what went well and repeat those successes. Each small win built confidence and reinforced the behaviors I wanted to make permanent. Starting any new venture, including weight loss, can feel awkward or overwhelming. When I first began managing my day-to-day food choices, my decisions weren't perfect—but over time, as I experienced wins, I began to trust the process. I started making better choices automatically, responding to cravings in healthier ways, and seeing progress not just on the scale, but in how I felt physically and mentally.

Each focus point comes with a practical homework assignment designed to keep you actively thinking about the task throughout the week. These assignments help you stay engaged, build consistency, and translate what you learn into real, lasting habits. They also encourage reflection, accountability, and self-awareness, all of which are key to developing a sustainable lifestyle. Are you ready to meet the new you? Let's take this journey together—one step, one habit, and one small victory at a time.

There may be times when you experience a backslide and feel so overwhelmed that restarting seems impossible. How do you pick yourself up and get back on track? I often tell my patients to think like a toddler: toddlers fall many times before they finally stand and walk. Anytime we begin a new venture, we are not going to be perfect.

Often, fear of starting over comes from trying to do too much at once. I call this the "New Year's Eve phenomenon"—wanting to exercise daily, drink enough water, and prepare all meals perfectly starting Monday morning. It feels overwhelming, and instead of making progress, we accomplish nothing. The key is to start small. Focus on achievable, manageable changes. Begin by drinking enough water each day. Once that becomes routine, add another habit. Don't focus on the big picture all at once; it's the small, consistent actions every day that create long-term results.

If you've had a moment of overeating or feel off track, return to your meal plan template and follow it for your next meal. Pull out your "wire list" and repeat your five "whys" aloud—sometimes multiple times a day. This is not a one-time exercise; it's a tool to help you remain mindful and intentional with your choices. Food can be addictive, whether society wants to acknowledge it or not. Like alcohol or drugs, it occupies our thoughts daily—but unlike substances, we must find a balance. That's why it's essential to use your tools consistently every day.

Celebrate every win, no matter how small. Even one compliant meal can create momentum. One meal turns into two, then a full day, and eventually, the scale begins moving in the right direction. With each success, you build confidence in your ability to complete tasks and reinforce the behaviors that lead to lasting weight loss.

By following these focus points, applying the homework assignments, and embracing the small, incremental changes, you are creating a foundation for sustainable health. This is a journey of growth, reflection, and empowerment—and each step forward brings you closer to the person you are capable of becoming.

Quote *Nothing changes if nothing changes.*

Focus 1. What is your commitment level

Understanding your commitment level helps you set achievable weight loss goals and avoid frustration or feelings of failure. Being honest with yourself reduces the chances of giving up when challenges arise. Knowing your limits allows you to pace yourself and maintain balance throughout the process.

We all lead busy lives and juggle multiple responsibilities, but your commitment to lifestyle change must hold equal importance. With health comes longevity — and the ability to show up fully for your family, friends, and loved ones. If your plate is already too full, recognize that you may not be able to give 100% to this process right now, and that's okay. Awareness is the first step toward meaningful change.

Homework Assignment

Rate your commitment level on a scale of 0–10 (0 = no commitment, 10 = fully committed) and take time to reflect on that number. What does it reveal about your readiness and capacity to prioritize your health at this time?

Quote *"He who has a why to live can bear almost any how."*

Focus 2. Pursue Your Goals: Discover Your "Why"

Identify the goals that genuinely matter to you — whether it's improving your health, boosting your energy, or feeling more confident. Aligning your actions with your personal motivations makes the journey more rewarding and sustainable over time.

Place the same emphasis on your weight loss journey as you did when you were graduating from high school, earning your degree, completing a certification, or building a relationship with your significant other. You dedicate time to what matters most — and your health deserves that same level of importance.

Your "WHY" statement is one of the most powerful tools you can develop. It becomes your anchor when you encounter temptation or peer pressure — like when you're at a party and someone insists you "just have one bite." In those moments, knowing your "WHY" helps you stand firm in your commitment and make choices that align with your goals.

Examples of my Personal "WHYs":

- I want to shop at any store and wear clothes that fit comfortably.
- I want to see my collarbones and hands — signs that represent health and strength to me.
- I want to cross my legs easily without struggling.
- I want to protect myself from developing diabetes, high blood pressure, or joint pain caused by excess weight.
- I want to prove to myself that I can finish what I start — just like I did when I began running.

This isn't something to rush. It may take a week or two to complete. Don't try to sit down and finish it in one session. Instead, reflect as you go about your day. Whenever you think, "I wish I could fit into this outfit," or "I want to be a better example for my family," write it down.

Once you've gathered most of your reasons, rewrite them neatly in your own handwriting. Then, take a photo and save it as your phone wallpaper or keep copies where you'll see them often. You always have your phone with you — use it as a reminder of your purpose.

When you find yourself in a compromising situation, read five of your "WHYs" out loud. This isn't a one-time exercise. Every time the desire to give in resurfaces, repeat the process. Over time, this practice will strengthen your resolve and shift your mindset.

If it's not written in your own handwriting, it's easy to argue that you didn't truly write it. Make it personal. Make it real. The first time may feel awkward or forced — that's okay. The more you practice, the stronger and more automatic this mental tool becomes.

Homework Assignment

Write your detailed "WHY" statement over the next one to two weeks. When complete, rewrite it by hand, take a photo, and place it somewhere visible — or make it your phone background. Practice reading five "WHYs" aloud anytime temptation or doubt arises.

Quote *"Your health is your greatest wealth. Your health is an investment, not an expense."*

Focus 3. Getting Mentally and Physically Prepared for Lifestyle Changes

Preparing for lifestyle changes is both mental and physical. Mentally, it's about getting your mind ready for a new way of thinking and being open to learning different approaches. This means letting go of the "all or nothing" mentality and understanding that growth requires flexibility and patience.

Physically, change often happens one step at a time. Fitness and movement don't need to be extreme to be effective — even walking is a powerful form of exercise that supports weight loss, improves mood, and builds momentum. Start small, stay consistent, and celebrate progress along the way.

To set yourself up for success, plan and prepare. Approach your journey with a positive, growth-oriented mindset. Expect challenges, but view them as opportunities to learn, adapt, and strengthen your commitment. This process is not about perfection — it's about progress and creating habits that will last. I started with simple walks around my neighborhood before committing to intense workouts, which built confidence and consistency.

Homework Assignment

Clean your home of all tempting food items that could derail your progress. Create an environment that supports your goals and makes healthy choices the easy choices.

***Quote** "Be the best version of you."*

Focus 4. Small Changes

Setting SMART goals—Specific, Measurable, Achievable, Relevant, and Time-bound—helps you stay focused and realistic. Avoid setting goals that feel overwhelming; instead, start with small, attainable steps that build momentum over time.

A **SMART goal** is a structured approach to goal setting that helps make objectives clear, achievable, and measurable. The acronym **SMART** stands for:

- **S – Specific:** The goal clearly defines what you want to accomplish.

-
- **M – Measurable:** It includes a way to track progress and know when success has been achieved.

- **A – Achievable:** The goal is realistic and within your ability or resources to accomplish.

- **R – Relevant:** It aligns with your personal values, needs, and long-term objectives.

- **T – Time-bound:** It has a clear timeline or deadline for completion.

When applied to **weight loss**, SMART goals transform vague intentions into actionable plans. Instead of saying, *"I want to lose weight,"* a SMART goal might be, *"I will lose 10 pounds in the next 8 weeks by walking 30 minutes five days per week and tracking my meals daily."*

Here's how SMART goals benefit weight loss:

1. **Clarity and focus:** They eliminate ambiguity, helping you know exactly what you're working toward.
2. **Motivation and accountability:** Breaking big goals into smaller, measurable steps creates steady progress and boosts confidence.
3. **Realistic expectations:** SMART goals prevent burnout and frustration by keeping goals attainable and aligned with your lifestyle.
4. **Consistency:** Setting a clear timeline encourages regular action rather than sporadic effort.
5. **Self-awareness:** Tracking progress promotes reflection, allowing you to identify what's working and where adjustments are needed.

In weight loss, SMART goals are powerful because they shift the focus from *"trying to lose weight"* to *"actively creating habits that lead to success."* This method builds structure, momentum, and a greater sense of control. (Bahrami et al.,2022)

For example, one simple and effective SMART goal is drinking more water. Research shows that when you are adequately hydrated, you're less likely to confuse thirst with hunger. Ideally, you should drink at least half your body weight in ounces of water daily.

For me, that's about 77.5 ounces, since I weigh 155 pounds. To make this goal easier to achieve, I use a 40-ounce cup and aim to drink two full cups per day. Thinking of it as "two cups" feels much more manageable than tracking several smaller bottles of water.

Homework Assignment

Identify one small, realistic task to focus on for the remaining weeks—such as adding an extra vegetable to your meals, taking a short walk after lunch, or increasing your daily water intake. Small changes lead to lasting results.

Quote *"For a seed to achieve its greatest expression, it must come completely undone. The shell cracks, its insides come out, and everything changes. To someone who doesn't understand growth, it would look like complete destruction."*

—*Cynthia Occelli*

Focus 5. Inner Change for Long-Term Results

There are three levels to changing behavior:

1. Identity
2. Process
3. Outcomes

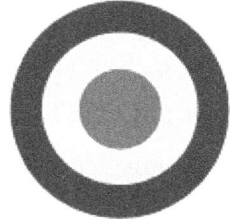

levels of changing behavior, picture these levels like a bullseye—with identity at the center, process in the middle layer, and outcomes on the outer ring. Changing one's identity means shifting your beliefs, self-image, and how one sees oneself. The process involves the daily actions and routines that help you reach your goals. The outcomes are the visible results you want—such as weight loss or improved fitness.

When change is focused only on outcomes, habits tend to be short-lived. For example, someone might lose weight temporarily but still see themselves as "overweight." Because their identity hasn't changed, old habits often return, and the progress fades.

The deepest and most powerful change happens at the level of identity. When you begin to believe, "I am a healthy person," your actions start to align with that belief. You naturally make better food choices, prioritize movement, and become more mindful of your overall health. This kind of transformation is ongoing—it's a lifelong process of becoming the person you aspire to be (Clear, 2018). Shift your thinking from outcome-based to identity-based habits. Don't let the scale define your success—let your daily choices and consistent habits do that. People who focus on identity act in alignment with who they believe they are.

Homework Assignment

Reflect—
- Who am I?
- Who do I want to become?

An identity-based individual focuses on building healthy habits and becoming that new version of themselves—regardless of what the scale says.

An outcome-based individual focuses only on results and may feel frustrated when progress slows, which often leads to rebound weight gain and discouragement.

Putting It All Together. Redefining Success Beyond the Scale

A 60-year-old woman has been following the program for several months and continues to measure her success solely by the number on the scale. When the scale goes down, she feels accomplished and proud. But when it doesn't move—or worse, when it goes up a pound or two—she becomes discouraged and reacts by skipping meals, thinking that eating less will make the weight come off faster. How could she improve her outcomes?

She could begin to shift her mindset from scale-focused to habit-focused. Her true progress comes from consistency and daily habits, not just the daily number on the scale.

Let's review the patterns that need improvement.

1. **Skipping Meals:**

   By skipping meals, she is slowing her metabolism and causing her body to hold onto fat instead of burning it. Her energy dips, and she becomes hungrier later in the day, which leads to overeating or poor food choices.

2. **Lack of Balanced Nutrition:**

   Without consistent protein intake throughout the day, her muscle mass is decreasing, which can make the scale number misleading. She may lose water or muscle rather than fat.

3. **Mindset and Emotional Triggers:**

Her emotional connection to the scale drives her behaviors instead of her long-term goals. She needs to redefine what "success" looks like—progress in energy, mood, sleep, and clothing fit are just as important as the number.

Focus points to review:

- Know What You Are Eating: Track meals consistently, not to restrict, but to ensure she's fueling her body with balanced nutrition.
- Understanding Macros: Keep her protein intake steady throughout the day to maintain lean muscle and support fat loss.
- Mindset and "Why": Focus on her "why"—to stay healthy, active, and strong as she ages. She begins journaling non-scale victories, like having more energy, less joint pain, or better sleep.
- Consistency Over Perfection: The provider reminds her that weight naturally fluctuates. What matters most is sticking to healthy habits over time.

Within a few weeks, she notices she feels more satisfied, her energy levels are stable, and her clothes fit better—even when the scale doesn't always drop. She begins to understand that eating the right foods consistently supports long-term results, while skipping meals only works against her goals.

By shifting her focus from the scale to the process, she finally starts building a healthier, more balanced relationship with food—and with herself.

Quote *"We are not what we know but what we are willing to learn."*

Focus 6. What Is Your Eating Style?

Choose an eating plan you can maintain for life. Avoid crash diets that promise quick results but are difficult to sustain long-term. Prioritize consistency over intensity—lasting results come from steady habits, not short bursts of extreme restriction. The best eating plan is one that fits seamlessly into your lifestyle and supports your health goals.

Many people begin their weight loss journey by following trends they've seen on social media or copying what worked for a friend. While these methods might bring short-term results for some, they often fail because the individual doesn't fully understand the plan or how it works. Knowledge is power—understanding the why and how behind your eating style helps you stay consistent and make informed choices.

It's important to remember that there is no one-size-fits-all diet. What works for someone else may not work for you, and that's okay. The key is to find a balanced approach that feels sustainable, enjoyable, and aligned with your personal goals.

Homework Assignment

Identify and understand the eating style you are following.

- What are its main principles?
- What foods are encouraged or limited?
- Does it align with your lifestyle and health needs?

People who take the time to fully understand their chosen approach are more likely to succeed and less likely to become frustrated when progress differs from others. The goal isn't to follow a specific diet—it's to create a lifestyle of eating that you can maintain long-term.

Focus 7. What Is Your Weakness?

Recognizing your triggers and obstacles is key to long-term success. These challenges may be emotional (stress, boredom), environmental (certain foods in the house), or situational (social gatherings, celebrations). Awareness allows you to prepare for these moments and manage them effectively instead of reacting impulsively.

It's rare for someone to truly not know what triggers their moments of weakness. Often, we do know—we just may not stop to reflect before acting. For example, a personal trigger for me is Reese's cups. I absolutely love them, and if they're in the house, they might as well already be eaten! During my weight loss journey, I learned not to buy them because having them around would sabotage my progress. Instead, I would plan to enjoy one during my monthly cheat meal, rather than giving in to the craving in the moment.

By recognizing and acknowledging the foods or situations that tempt you, you can make conscious decisions that support your goals. This doesn't mean you can never have your favorite treats—it simply means being strategic and intentional about when and how you enjoy them.

Homework Assignment

Identify one trigger that challenges you.

- What situations or emotions cause you to veer off track?
- How can you plan ahead to manage or avoid that trigger?
- What healthier alternative or coping strategy can you use instead?

Take the time to reflect and make a personal commitment to avoid keeping your trigger foods or situations within easy reach. There will always be a time and place to enjoy your favorite treats, but while building new habits, it's important to set yourself up for success by minimizing temptation.

Quote *The one who falls and gets up is stronger than the one who never tried.*

Focus 8. Learn from Your Setbacks

What is a setback?

A setback is any moment when you fall off track from your weight loss plan—whether it's skipping workouts, overeating, or emotional eating. Setbacks are a normal part of any lifestyle change and happen to everyone at some point. They don't mean you've failed; they simply signal that something needs adjusting.

Why it's important to face them

Dealing with setbacks during weight loss is one of the most important parts of creating a sustainable and healthy relationship with food, movement, and yourself. The way you respond to those moments determines your long-term success. When setbacks happen, take time to examine what caused them and how you can prevent them in the future. Instead of seeing them as failures, view them as opportunities to grow stronger and refine your approach.

I struggled with this area myself because of my "all-or-nothing" mentality. Whenever I gave in to temptation, I felt frustrated and defeated. I'd tell myself, "Oh well, I already had one bad meal—might as well eat whatever I want for the rest of the day." Unfortunately, that "day" often turned into weeks before I found my way back on track.

Through my own research and experience, I learned the importance of reflecting instead of reacting. When I took time to pause and understand what triggered the setback—stress, fatigue, or lack of planning—I was able to make better choices the next time. Reflection helped me shift from a mindset of punishment to one of learning and resilience. It taught me that one slip doesn't erase all progress; it simply offers a chance to reset and move forward with more awareness.

When I slipped up, I began asking myself:

- What caused this setback?
- Was I unprepared and didn't have my meals ready?
- Was I bored with my food choices?
- Was I stressed, tired, or emotionally drained?

By identifying the true cause, I could make practical changes instead of beating myself up. I also discovered something powerful—one bad day doesn't ruin your progress. When I got back on track immediately, the scale barely moved. But when I let a few days or weeks pass, the weight gain was noticeable.

Learning from your setbacks increases your self-awareness and builds resilience. Each time you reflect and adjust, you strengthen the habits that lead to lasting success.

Homework Assignment

Reflect on a recent setback you've experienced—whether related to food, exercise, or consistency. Write down what triggered it, how you responded, and what you could do differently next time. End your reflection with one positive takeaway that you can use to move forward.

Remember, setbacks don't define you—your response to them does. Progress is not about perfection; it's about getting back up, learning the lesson, and moving forward with more wisdom and strength.

Quote *"Success is the sum of small efforts, repeated day in and day out."*

—*Robert Collier*

Focus 9. The Three Pillars to Weight Loss Success

Sustainable weight loss is built on three key pillars: nutrition, hydration, and movement. These foundational habits work together to support your metabolism, energy levels, and long-term success.

1. Nutrition

One of the most common pitfalls is skipping meals, especially breakfast. While it may seem like an easy way to cut calories, skipping meals often leads to overeating later in the day. Aim for balanced meals that include lean protein, fiber-rich carbohydrates, and minimal fats to keep your energy steady and prevent cravings.

Remember, 80% of weight loss comes from nutrition. Not preparing your meals sets you up for failure. Take the time to plan ahead—either by cooking your own meals, using a meal prep company, or purchasing ready-made healthy options from your local grocery store. Having a Plan B is just as important: keep a few healthy, pre-prepared meals on hand for those times when you're tired, busy, or simply bored with your usual menu. Consistency and preparation are the true keys to success.

2. Hydration

Water plays a vital role in metabolism, appetite regulation, and overall health. Staying hydrated can help you distinguish between true hunger and thirst, supporting better food choices. Aim to drink water consistently throughout the day—about half of your body weight in ounces daily is a good starting point.

3. Movement

Physical activity supports weight management, improves mood, and strengthens the body. The American Heart Association (AHA) recommends 20–30 minutes of activity per day or reaching 10,000 steps daily. Choose a movement that you enjoy—walking, strength training, dancing, or any form of exercise that feels sustainable.

Homework Assignment

Reflect: *Which pillar do you need the most help with?*
- Nutrition
- Hydration
- Movement

You don't need to master all three pillars at once. Start by focusing on your weakest area and build consistency there. As you gain confidence and stability, gradually incorporate the other pillars. The more you integrate these practices into your daily life, the stronger your new habits will become.

Quote *"Let food be thy medicine and medicine be thy food."*

—Hippocrates.

Focus 10. Know What You Are Eating

Treat your food choices like managing a bank account—track your "spending" and stay intentional. When you journal what you eat, even briefly, you begin to recognize patterns and make more mindful decisions.

Most people who balance their checking accounts know exactly what's in the bank down to the penny and make decisions accordingly. Treat your food the same way. If a food is high in fat or calories, enjoy it in small portions and be aware of what you're consuming. Take a moment to read the nutrition label and understand what's actually going into your body. You wouldn't blindly spend money—so why spend calories without knowing the cost? After all, your body is far more valuable than your bank account.

When I started paying attention to the fat content in foods—especially nuts, cheeses, and wings (my personal favorites)—I was shocked. It felt like I had been overspending without checking my balance! Let's just say I didn't like the "account balance" reflected on the scale after a few weeks of those choices. That was my wake-up call to pay closer attention to what I was consuming and how quickly those calories added up.

Homework Assignment

Keep a simple food journal for three days. Write down everything you eat and drink, including snacks and condiments. Afterward, review your notes and look for patterns—times you eat out of habit, boredom, or stress, or foods that might be sneaking in extra calories. Identify one change you can make this week to be more intentional with your "spending."

Scenario—Putting it all together

A 50-year-old woman has reached a point in her journey where she is frustrated. She has not been as consistent with her eating or movement as she was in the beginning. She says, "I don't know why I'm not losing weight—I've been following the plan, but the scale hasn't moved."

Let's review where she may need reinforcement.

Portion Creep: Over time, her portion sizes have slowly increased. She hasn't been measuring her food as carefully and has started eyeballing servings, which has led to consuming more calories than she realizes.

Protein Intake: She's been skipping some meals or relying on quick snacks, resulting in lower protein intake and higher fat or carb consumption. This imbalance is affecting her metabolism and satiety.

1. **Movement:** Her exercise routine has become inconsistent. She used to walk 30 minutes daily but has recently missed several days due to her schedule.
2. **Mindfulness and Tracking:** She stopped journaling her meals and isn't fully aware of what or how much she's eating.

Focus Points to Review

- **Know What You Are Eating:** Begin journaling meals again and track all food intake for awareness and accountability.
- **Understanding Macros:** Reassess her balance—aim for approximately 40% protein, 40% carbohydrates, and 20% fat to support fat loss and lean muscle preservation.

- **<u>Movement:</u>** Recommit to 20–30 minutes of daily physical activity, even if it's walking or light resistance training. (Use the habit tracker to remind her of her commitment)
- **<u>Mindset and Consistency:</u>** Revisit her "why" statements to strengthen motivation and refocus her mental commitment to long-term habits.

After implementing these focus points again, she begins to see progress. Within a few weeks, her energy improves, her clothes fit better, and the scale begins to move. The key to breaking her stall wasn't a drastic change—it was returning to the basics with intention and consistency.

Quote _"Time and health are two precious assets that we don't recognize until they're depleted."_

Focus 11. Understanding Macros

Protein, fat, and carbohydrates each play vital roles in your body. Protein supports muscle repair and helps you feel full; fat nourishes your brain and hormones, and carbohydrates provide the energy your body needs to function at its best.

Every eating plan has its own macro balance. For example, when you're cutting for fat loss, your diet will typically include less fat and more protein. On the other hand, a ketogenic diet focuses on high fat and very low carbohydrates. Understanding the macro structure of your chosen eating plan helps you follow it correctly and achieve the results you want.

If you're following the Habit-Based Weight Loss Meal Plan, reflect on your compliance. Are you truly hitting your macro goals?

Homework Assignment

Track your daily intake and ensure your macros are around 40% protein, 40% carbohydrates, and 20% fat.

Quote *"Let's build wellness rather than treat disease."*

Focus 12. How to Handle Holidays, Vacations, and Busy Schedules

Plan ahead so you can enjoy special occasions without guilt. Stay hydrated, keep your body moving, and practice flexibility. Life will always bring holidays, trips, and busy days—success comes from focusing on progress, not perfection.

These moments can be challenging, but with planning, you can enjoy them without gaining weight. Continue to follow your usual structure of eating six times a day. When attending a celebration or event, aim to consume the same portion sizes as you would at home. You don't need to bring a food scale—

just use your best judgment to "eyeball" portions of protein, starches, and carbs.

The main goal during these events is maintenance—to enjoy yourself while staying in control and keeping your progress intact. Remember, it's absolutely possible to have fun and still maintain your weight.

Homework Assignment

Write out your personal strategy for navigating holidays, vacations, or busy work schedules while staying on track with your health goals.

Scenario

A 40-year-old woman is preparing for a week-long family vacation. She's worked hard to lose weight and feels great in her progress, but she knows vacations can be filled with tempting, calorie-dense foods and less structure. Her goal is to maintain her weight during the trip, not to lose more, but to prove to herself that she can enjoy life while staying consistent.

Before leaving, she reviews her focus points—meal planning, hydration, daily movement, mindfulness, and remembering her "why." She reminds herself that her "why" is to feel confident, energetic, and in control of her health so she can be active with her family and not feel sluggish or regretful afterward.

During the trip, her family goes out for breakfast, lunch, and dinner each day. Pancakes, burgers, and desserts are everywhere. Instead of feeling deprived, she uses her tools. She eats small, portioned meals every few hours, bringing protein snacks with her like boiled eggs, turkey jerky, and protein shakes. When offered calorie-dense foods, she pauses and silently repeats five of her "why" statements to keep her mindset strong. This helps her say no to overeating and yes to moderation.

She still enjoys the vacation—she has a few bites of dessert, shares appetizers, and enjoys local meals—but she practices awareness and balance. She drinks plenty of water, walks daily with her family, and stays mindful of her hunger cues.

By the end of the week, she feels proud and empowered. She didn't gain weight, didn't feel restricted, and most importantly, she proved that the habits she built truly work. Her focus points—planning, mindfulness, portion control, and remembering her "why"—helped her stay consistent and confident throughout her vacation.

Quote _"The greatest mistake you can make in life is to be continually fearing you will make one."_

Focus 13. Preparing for Maintenance

Maintenance is not the end of your journey—it's the continuation of your healthy lifestyle. It requires consistent effort, awareness, and reflection. Regularly check in with your goals and keep practicing the habits that helped you succeed in the first place.

There shouldn't be a big difference between weight loss and maintenance because whatever you do to lose weight is what you'll need to do to keep it off. Many people struggle because their weight loss plan was overly restrictive— something they couldn't sustain long-term. When that happens, even small setbacks can make it hard to regain control.

To make maintenance successful, focus on sustainability. Build a routine that fits your real life and supports your long-term well-being. Think back on the Pillars of Weight Loss Success:

- Drinking 80 oz of water daily
- Meal prepping and planning
- Moving your body for 20–30 minutes daily

Ask yourself—is there one pillar you still need to strengthen? Use this insight to create an action plan for lasting success.

Homework Assignment

Identify the areas in your routine that still need improvement and outline how you'll strengthen them moving forward.

Quote *"Repetition is the mother of learning, the father of action, which makes it the architect of accomplishment."*

Focus 14. Repeat and Refocus

Lifestyle change takes time, consistency, and repetition. Revisit these focus points as often as needed to strengthen your habits and mindset. Each time you repeat the process, you reinforce the foundation for long-term success.

Reaching your goal weight isn't the end of the journey—it's simply a new phase. Maintenance and continued progress require the same daily habits that helped you get here. The tools, strategies, and focus points you've learned are meant to be used over and over until they become second nature.

Think of it like managing a lifelong condition—just as someone with diabetes must always stay mindful of their food choices, you'll always need to stay aware of what you're eating, how much, and why. This awareness isn't a burden—it's a form of empowerment that keeps you in control of your health and results.

When challenges arise, refocus on what you know works: your habits, your structure, and your "why." Consistency—not perfection—is what keeps you successful.

Homework Assignment

Review your journey so far. Celebrate how far you've come, and set new goals for your next phase of growth.

What if I'm Not Ready or I Fail

Are you feeling overwhelmed or unsure if you can be successful on this journey? I understand—so did I. For anyone feeling this way, it's important to understand the concept of the program, but it must be simplified into a form that is achievable. Instead of trying to tackle everything at once, begin with the one area you may need the most help with. Think back on the three pillars for successful weight loss and maintenance: drinking 80 ounces of water daily, meal prepping and planning, or 20–30 minutes of movement each day. Which one feels the most challenging for you? Start there. The key is to focus on building small, sustainable habits rather than attempting a full-scale lifestyle overhaul all at once.

Remember your first day of school, your first day at work, or the first time you learned to ride a bike. You did not start out like a pro. You may have failed an exam, made a mistake at work, or fallen off the bike. You did not give up—you kept at it. Eventually, it became second nature. The same principle applies to habit-based weight loss.

Begin by increasing awareness of your current habits. Keep a simple diary for two to three days, noting meals, snacks, beverages, and physical activity. Look for patterns, such as times when unhealthy habits are triggered by stress, boredom, or social situations. It's also important to acknowledge and validate your feelings of overwhelm, and remember that meaningful change is gradual, not instant.

Next, choose one small, achievable habit to focus on first. Examples could include drinking 16–20 ounces of water first thing in the morning, adding one serving of vegetables to lunch or dinner, or taking a ten-minute walk after lunch. Setting a goal that is specific, measurable, achievable, relevant, and time-bound helps keep your efforts realistic and trackable.

Identify your barriers and triggers. Consider environmental factors, like keeping unhealthy foods at home, and emotional triggers, such as stress eating or boredom. Develop strategies to prevent these triggers from derailing your progress, such as keeping Plan B meals available, practicing mindfulness, or using distraction techniques.

Focus on identity-based change by thinking about who you want to become rather than solely what you want to achieve. Shift your attention from outcomes, like the number on the scale, to daily actions that reflect a healthy self-image. For example, instead of saying, "I want to lose 20 pounds," try, "I am someone who makes balanced food choices."

Build a simple routine by starting with manageable, repeatable actions. Avoid trying to implement too many changes at once and emphasize consistency over perfection.

Use accountability and support to strengthen your habits. Track your progress with checklists, apps, or journaling, and seek encouragement from family, friends, or support groups. Celebrate small wins along the way to build confidence and motivation.

Plan for setbacks by recognizing that occasional lapses are a normal part of the process and valuable learning opportunities, not failures. Reflect on what triggered the setback and develop a plan to prevent it in the future. Maintaining a growth mindset helps reinforce that progress comes from consistency, not speed.

Ultimately, the focus should be on small, sustainable, identity-based habits rather than perfection. By taking clear, simple steps, anticipating challenges, and committing to steady progress, you set yourself up for long-term success.

Additional Scenarios

These scenarios are real-life situations I have encountered repeatedly over the years. I've put together practical tools designed to help you navigate whatever challenges or setbacks you may face on your journey. Take a moment to reflect—do any of these resonate with you? Explore the strategies I recommend to help you work through your most challenging situations and move forward with confidence.

Scenario: Building Structure in a Busy Schedule

A 35-year-old man comes to his first appointment ready to start his weight loss journey. He explains that his biggest challenge is his demanding work schedule. His days are packed with back-to-back meetings, long commutes, and little time for breaks. He often skips breakfast and lunch, then eats one large meal late at night. He knows this pattern isn't healthy, but doesn't see how he can fit smaller meals into his day.

The provider helps him understand that skipping meals slows his metabolism, increases hunger, and leads to overeating later. Together, they identify ways he can use the focus points to build structure and consistency even with a busy lifestyle:

1. **Plan and Prepare (Know What You Are Eating):**
    He commits to meal prepping twice a week—on Sundays and Wednesdays. He prepares quick, portable meals like hard-boiled eggs, turkey roll-ups, protein shakes, Greek yogurt, and pre-portioned nuts. This ensures he always has balanced options ready to grab and go.

2. **Eat Small, Frequent Meals:**
    The provider suggests setting reminders on his phone every 3–4 hours to prompt him to eat something small. Even a protein bar, shake, or handful of almonds can help keep his metabolism active and prevent overeating later.

3. **Hydration and Mindfulness:**
    He starts carrying a large reusable water bottle to meetings. Staying hydrated helps control hunger and maintain energy levels throughout the day.

4. **Understanding Macros:**
    He learns that eating protein with every meal helps him stay full and supports fat loss. He aims for balanced macros around 40% protein, 40% carbohydrates, and 20% fat.

5. **Movement:**
    Since his schedule is tight, he incorporates short bursts of movement—taking the stairs, parking farther away, or doing a quick 10-minute walk between meetings.

These small actions add up and support his overall progress.

6. **Mindset and Consistency:**
   He reminds himself of his "why"—to feel more energetic, improve his health, and be a positive example for his family. Focusing on his purpose helps him stay consistent even when work gets stressful.

Within a few weeks, he notices that his energy levels are higher, his cravings are under control, and he's no longer ravenous at night. The structure created through the focus points helps him realize that even with a busy schedule, small, intentional changes make a big difference. His success comes not from having more time, but from using the time he has with purpose and planning.

Scenario: Balancing Family Life While Staying Committed to Goals

A 34-year-old woman wants to lose weight and improve her health. She's motivated, but her husband isn't interested in making dietary changes, and their two children are involved in multiple sports activities. Evenings are chaotic—between practices, games, and quick dinners on the go, she often ends up eating whatever is convenient. She tells her provider, "I feel like I'm cooking different meals for everyone, and I just don't have the time."

The provider helps her see that success doesn't mean cooking separate meals—it means learning how to plan, prepare, and adapt using the program's focus points so her choices fit naturally into family life.

1. **Plan Ahead and Keep It Simple (Know What You Are Eating):**
   She starts by planning family meals that can work for everyone. For example, she cooks grilled chicken, roasted vegetables, and rice. Her husband and kids can add sauces or sides they enjoy, while she measures her portions to stay on track. This way, everyone eats the same base meal without her feeling like a short-order cook.

2. **Meal Prep and Portioning:**
   On Sundays, she preps proteins like chicken, ground turkey, and boiled eggs, and stores them in containers. She also chops vegetables and preps grab-and-go snacks for busy evenings. This allows her to make quick, healthy meals even when the family is running out the door.

3. **Hydration and Mindful Choices:**
   She carries a water bottle and focuses on staying hydrated during the day. When eating out at her kids' games or grabbing food on the go, she looks for simple options—grilled proteins, side salads, or fruit cups instead of fried foods or sugary snacks.

4. **Understanding Macros:**
   She aims for balanced meals with lean protein, moderate carbs, and healthy fats (around 40/40/20%). If the family is having pizza night, she enjoys one slice with a large salad or extra veggies to keep her macros balanced while still participating.

5. **Movement and Consistency:**
   Instead of trying to find a full hour for workouts, she walks around the field during her kids' practices or does short home workouts in the morning. Small, consistent activity adds up.

6. **Mindset and Her "Why":**
   When tempted to give up or feel frustrated, she reminds herself of her "why"—to have more energy, feel confident, and set an example for her children. She focuses on progress, not perfection.

After a few weeks, she realizes that she doesn't need to make completely separate meals. By preparing versatile foods, managing portions, and planning ahead, she feels in control and less stressed. Her family still enjoys their favorite meals, and she stays on track with her goals. She's no longer a short-order cook—she's a role model showing her family what balanced, healthy living looks like in real life.

Scenario: Understanding That Medication Is a Tool, Not the Solution

A 46-year-old patient comes in for a follow-up visit, feeling proud of her progress. She's lost 25 pounds since starting her weight loss medication and says, "This medication is amazing—I don't even have to try that hard. It's doing all the work for me."

Her provider congratulates her on her progress but gently explains that while the medication is helping, it's not the reason she's losing weight—it's the tool that's allowing her to make better lifestyle choices. The provider reminds her that the true success comes from how she's been eating, planning, and building healthier habits.

They review her habits and discuss where the real progress has been made:

1. **Appetite Control, Not Magic:**
   The medication helps reduce her appetite, which gives her the space to make smarter food choices—but she's the one choosing what to eat. The scale is moving because she's fueling her body better, not starving it.

2. **Structure and Focus Points:**
   She has been following the program—eating six small meals a day, prioritizing protein, staying hydrated, and moving regularly. These behaviors are what drive fat

loss and metabolic health. The medication simply helps make them easier to follow.

3. **Long-Term Reality:**

   The provider explains that medication is often temporary or adjusted over time. When it's stopped, if she hasn't built consistent habits, the weight will return. Lifestyle change is what ensures lasting results.

To reinforce this, the provider revisits key focus points with her:

Know What You Are Eating: Continue journaling and reading nutrition labels to stay aware of food choices.

Understanding Macros: Keep meals balanced—around 40% protein, 40% carbs, and 20% fat—to preserve lean muscle and prevent rebound weight gain.

Hydration: Maintain consistent water intake, as dehydration can slow results and trigger cravings.

- Movement: Exercise supports metabolism and keeps weight off long-term.

Mindset and "Why": Remember that the medication is a stepping stone—it's her effort and consistency that create transformation.

After reflecting, she realizes how much her habits have changed since starting the program. She now preps meals, eats balanced portions, walks daily, and drinks water regularly—all things she didn't do before.

Her provider tells her, "The medication opened the door, but you're the one walking through it."

Over time, as she continues to apply the focus points, she begins to see herself—not the medication—as the true reason behind her success. The shift in mindset gives her confidence that she can maintain her progress with or without medication because she's built the skills and structure to support lifelong health.

Scenario: Learning to Use All the Focus Points

A 52-year-old man has been on the weight loss program for a few weeks, but is frustrated. He admits that he only uses the focus points he likes and ignores the rest. He says, "I don't see how these apply to me. I just pick and choose what's convenient, and nothing is changing."

The provider explains that the focus points are not optional—they work as a system. Skipping one or two can block progress because each supports a different part of weight loss and habit building. The key is learning how to incorporate them into daily life in a practical way.

1. **Know What You Are Eating:**
   The provider shows him how journaling meals for just a few minutes a day can reveal hidden habits—like snacking late at night or eating larger portions than

intended. He starts by taking photos of meals or logging quick notes instead of spending hours tracking.

2. **Understanding Macros:**
He learns that paying attention to protein, carbs, and fats isn't about perfection—it's about structure. By keeping his meals roughly balanced, he feels fuller longer and avoids cravings.

3. **Meal Planning and Prep:**
The provider helps him plan simple meals that can be repeated throughout the week. For example, grilled chicken, steamed vegetables, and brown rice can be prepped in bulk and easily portioned.

4. **Mindset and "Why":**
The provider guides him to identify his personal "why"—whether it's health, energy, or longevity. Repeating these statements daily strengthens commitment and motivation.

By integrating all the focus points—even in small, realistic ways—he begins to see results. For instance, journaling helps him notice late-night snacking, balanced meals reduce hunger between meals, and short bouts of movement improve energy. He learns that the focus points aren't separate tasks; they are interconnected tools that make sustainable change possible.

Within a few weeks, he feels more in control, less frustrated, and starts seeing steady progress on the scale. The key lesson: using the focus points together, even imperfectly, is far more effective than picking and choosing selectively.

Your journey starts now—take that first step with confidence. The tools, strategies, and focus points you've learned are not just temporary steps—they are the foundation for lasting habits, health, and self-assurance.

Throughout this book, you've seen how real people navigate life's challenges—vacations, busy schedules, family responsibilities, plateaus, and setbacks. Their circumstances may vary, but the principles remain the same: awareness, consistency, intentional choices, and a strong "why." These are your tools, and they work in any situation—if you choose to use them.

Sustainable weight loss and healthy living aren't about perfection, extremes, or quick fixes. They're about progress, reflection, and building a life that aligns with the person you want to become. Each focus point—from knowing what you eat and understanding macros, to planning meals, staying hydrated, moving regularly, and anchoring yourself in your "why"—works together to create a balanced, achievable approach.

You will face challenges. You will encounter setbacks. There will be days when frustration or overwhelm creeps in. That is normal. But every time you return to your focus points, reflect on your wins, and take intentional action, you strengthen your resilience, confidence, and commitment. Remember: one meal, one walk, one mindful choice can set the tone for an entire day—or even week—of progress.

Your journey is not defined by the number on the scale or temporary lapses. It is defined by your persistence, your choices, and your willingness to keep moving forward— especially when it feels hard. Every small step adds up. Every consistent action builds confidence. Every time you get back up after a setback, you prove to yourself that you can do this.

So, as you move forward, hold onto these truths:

- Stay consistent.
- Stay mindful.
- Stay patient.
- Celebrate your wins—big or small.
- Lean on your focus points—they are your roadmap.

You've learned the principles. You've seen them in action. You've practiced the tools. Now it's time to live them—every day—with purpose, pride, and confidence.

There are still moments when I look in the mirror or see myself in recent photos and mentally revert to the version of me that weighed over 200 pounds. You may experience this as well. Even after significant weight loss, the mind can hold onto an old image of the body long after the body has changed. When this happens, I remind myself that I am no longer that person. I return to my focus points and the daily habits that helped me lose the weight in the first place. These are the same habits that help me maintain it—while still living a life that feels enjoyable and balanced. There is a difference between being mindful of your health and slipping into extremes or disorder. I am not a mental health provider, but if you find that you are struggling to recognize or accept your new body, or if you begin restricting food out of fear of gaining weight, it may be helpful to speak with a counselor. This experience is often referred to as body dysmorphia or sometimes "phantom fat," where someone continues to see themselves as they once were, even when that image no longer matches reality (Ammenheuser, 2023). The important thing is to acknowledge those feelings with compassion, stay connected to your healthy habits, and seek support when needed.

No matter where you are in your journey, no matter how many times you've started over, remember this: you have everything you need to succeed. You are capable. You are strong. And yes—you can do it.

Your journey doesn't end here. It begins here, today, with the choices you make in this very moment. Take a step. Build a habit. Celebrate a win. And then do it again. One day at a time, you will create the life and health you've been working toward.

You've got this.

About the Author

Dr. Melissa Ramsey, DNP MSN, RN, FNP-C

Melissa Ramsey is a native of Maryland and a graduate of Towson State University. She began her career as a Coronary Care nurse at The University of Maryland Medical Center in Baltimore, where she spent seven years witnessing firsthand the effects of poor health. While working night shifts, she often spoke with patients recovering from heart attacks or awaiting transplants. Many would say, "If I could do life over again, I would have taken better care of my health."

These conversations inspired her passion for helping people achieve their health goals. She became certified as a group fitness instructor and personal trainer and holds certifications in Body Combat, Body Pump, Body Flow, and Warrior Strength.

In 2015, Mrs. Ramsey earned her master's degree from Bowie State University and joined Doctors Community Hospital as a breast cancer nurse practitioner, managing their high-risk program.

In 2020, she opened Get Your Body Back Wellness Center to support patients through habit-based weight loss. She is also a certified injector trained in injectables and body contouring. At the center, patients learn how to safely lose 1–2 pounds per week, adopt sustainable lifestyle changes, and celebrate milestones with pampering services.

Mrs. Ramsey is an active member of the American Association of Nurse Practitioners, Alpha Kappa Alpha Sorority, Incorporated, and Sigma Theta Tau International Nursing Honor Society.

She completed her Doctor of Nursing Practice (DNP) degree at Aspen University in 2023. Her dissertation, titled "Obesity: Strengthening Favorable Habits for Improved Adherence to Weight Loss Management," is available on ProQuest.

Dr. Melissa Ramsey actively sees patients in Maryland and accepts virtual or in-person appointments. Her license also allows her to see patients in California, Maryland, Alabama, DC, Oklahoma, Florida, Illinois, Iowa, Kansas, Tennessee, Utah, Texas, Virginia, North Carolina, Washington, and Minnesota.

Focus Point	Homework Assignment
Prep Week	Understanding the meal template, purchase a food scale and containers
What is your commitment level?	Homework assignment: rate your commitment level on a scale of (0-10), 0, meaning no commitment, to 10 fully committed, and self-reflect on that number
Pursue Your Goals: Identify your "WHY"	Homework Assignment: Write down your "Why?"
Getting Mentally and Physically Prepared for Lifestyle Changes:	Homework Assignment: Clean your house of all tempting food items.
Small Changes	Homework Assignment: Identify one small task to work on for the remaining weeks. *Receive a habit tracker.
Inner Change for long-term results	Homework Assignment: Who am I? Who do I want to become?
What is your eating style?	Homework assignment: Identify and fully understand the eating style you are following
What is your weakness?	Homework Assignment: Identify one trigger that challenges you.
Learn from your setbacks.	Homework Assignment: What did I learn from my most recent setback?

The 3 Pillars to Weight Loss Success	Homework: Which pillar do you need the most help with?
Know what you are eating	Document everything you eat + nutritional Information.
Understanding Macros	Homework Assignment: Are you keeping your macros at 40/40/20%?
How to handle travel, events, and celebrations	
Getting prepared for maintenance	Time to strengthen any weak focus points

Meal Plan Template

You must make changes to see different results! No one can do this for you.

Portion Guidelines

Protein Choices (≤5g fat per serving)

- Egg whites
- Boneless skinless chicken breast
- Boneless skinless turkey breast
- Lean ground beef
- 1% lean ground turkey
- Cod, Tuna, Seafood
- Tofu, Pork

Protein Portion Sizes

- Women: 4 oz
- Men: 6 oz

Carbohydrate Choices (Items included in this category are starchy vegetables/grains/fruit)

- Rolled or steel-cut oats
- Quinoa

- Brown rice
- Yams/Sweet potato
- Bread
- Fruit (Any fruit)
- Corn, Carrots, Peas, Edamame, Beans, Brussels sprouts

Carbohydrate Portion Sizes

- Women: 2 oz
  Men: 3 oz

Non-Starchy Vegetables (Unlimited)

- Broccoli, Asparagus, Kale, Spinach
- Onions, Tomatoes, Garlic, Lettuce, Cabbage, Salad

Fat Guidelines

- 40% carbs, 40% protein, 20% fat
- Minimize eating out (too calorie-dense or high-fat) for the first 30 days
- Do not add/consume: oils, butter, mayo, oil sprays, margarine, peanut/nut butters, cheese, hummus, avocado, wings, or meat on the bone
- Use unlimited seasonings, herbs, or broth for flavor

Eating Schedule

- Eat every 3–4 hours
- Every meal must include:
- 1 portion protein
- 1 portion carb
- Unlimited non-starchy vegetables
- Alternate meals with a protein shake, bar, or baked lean meat if desired
- Drink ½ your body weight in ounces of water daily

Snack Rules

- High protein: 12–30g per snack
- Less than 5g fat per snack
- Options: Protein shakes/bars (Quest, Premier, Pure Protein, Ka'Chava), Greek yogurt, cottage cheese, deli meat

Sample Day Template

Meal 1

- Protein: _____ (4 oz Women/6 oz Men)

- Carbs: _____ (2 oz Women/3 oz Men)

- Non Starchy Vegetables: _____ (Unlimited)

Snack 1

- Protein source: _____

Meal 2

- Protein: _____

- Carbs: _____

- Non Starchy Vegetables: _____

Snack 2

- Protein source: _____

Meal 3

- Protein: _____

- Carbs: _____

- Non Starchy Vegetables: _____

Snack 3

- Protein source: _____

Tips for Success

- Prep meals ahead of time to stay on track during busy days.
- Alternate protein shakes or bars with lean meat to simplify meals.
- Use the open/closed hand method for portion control if a scale isn't available.
- Briefly track your meals to ensure you're hitting your protein, carb, and veggie goals.
- Read food labels and be mindful of the fat content. If the serving of fat is more than 5 grams of fat per serving. I recommend selecting something else.
- Celebrate small victories, like drinking enough water or hitting your protein goal for a snack.

Female Meal Tracker

MONDAY MEAL 1	MEAL 2	MEAL 3
☐ 4oz Lean Meat	☐ 4oz Lean Meat	☐ 4oz Lean Meat
☐ 3oz Starchy Veggie/Carbs	☐ 3oz Starchy Veggie/Carbs	☐ 3oz Starchy Veggie/Carbs
☐ **Unlimited** Non-Starchy Veggie	☐ **Unlimited** Non-Starchy Veggie	☐ **Unlimited** Non-Starchy Veggie
SNACK 1	**SNACK 2**	**SNACK 3**
☐ 12 - 30 Grams of Protein	☐ 12 - 30 Grams of Protein	☐ 12 - 30 Grams of Protein
☐ < 5 Grams of Fat	☐ < 5 Grams of Fat	☐ < 5 Grams of Fat

TUESDAY MEAL 1	MEAL 2	MEAL 3
☐ 4oz Lean Meat	☐ 4oz Lean Meat	☐ 4oz Lean Meat
☐ 3oz Starchy Veggie/Carbs	☐ 3oz Starchy Veggie/Carbs	☐ 3oz Starchy Veggie/Carbs
☐ **Unlimited** Non-Starchy Veggie	☐ **Unlimited** Non-Starchy Veggie	☐ **Unlimited** Non-Starchy Veggie
SNACK 1	**SNACK 2**	**SNACK 3**
☐ 12 - 30 Grams of Protein	☐ 12 - 30 Grams of Protein	☐ 12 - 30 Grams of Protein
☐ < 5 Grams of Fat	☐ < 5 Grams of Fat	☐ < 5 Grams of Fat

WEDNESDAY MEAL 1	MEAL 2	MEAL 3
☐ 4oz Lean Meat	☐ 4oz Lean Meat	☐ 4oz Lean Meat
☐ 3oz Starchy Veggie/Carbs	☐ 3oz Starchy Veggie/Carbs	☐ 3oz Starchy Veggie/Carbs
☐ **Unlimited** Non-Starchy Veggie	☐ **Unlimited** Non-Starchy Veggie	☐ **Unlimited** Non-Starchy Veggie
SNACK 1	**SNACK 2**	**SNACK 3**
☐ 12 - 30 Grams of Protein	☐ 12 - 30 Grams of Protein	☐ 12 - 30 Grams of Protein
☐ < 5 Grams of Fat	☐ < 5 Grams of Fat	☐ < 5 Grams of Fat

THURSDAY MEAL 1	MEAL 2	MEAL 3
☐ 4oz Lean Meat	☐ 4oz Lean Meat	☐ 4oz Lean Meat
☐ 3oz Starchy Veggie/Carbs	☐ 3oz Starchy Veggie/Carbs	☐ 3oz Starchy Veggie/Carbs
☐ **Unlimited** Non-Starchy Veggie	☐ **Unlimited** Non-Starchy Veggie	☐ **Unlimited** Non-Starchy Veggie
SNACK 1	**SNACK 2**	**SNACK 3**
☐ 12 - 30 Grams of Protein	☐ 12 - 30 Grams of Protein	☐ 12 - 30 Grams of Protein
☐ < 5 Grams of Fat	☐ < 5 Grams of Fat	☐ < 5 Grams of Fat

FRIDAY MEAL 1	MEAL 2	MEAL 3
☐ 4oz Lean Meat	☐ 4oz Lean Meat	☐ 4oz Lean Meat
☐ 3oz Starchy Veggie/Carbs	☐ 3oz Starchy Veggie/Carbs	☐ 3oz Starchy Veggie/Carbs
☐ **Unlimited** Non-Starchy Veggie	☐ **Unlimited** Non-Starchy Veggie	☐ **Unlimited** Non-Starchy Veggie
SNACK 1	SNACK 2	SNACK 3
☐ 12 - 30 Grams of Protein	☐ 12 - 30 Grams of Protein	☐ 12 - 30 Grams of Protein
☐ < 5 Grams of Fat	☐ < 5 Grams of Fat	☐ < 5 Grams of Fat

SATURDAY MEAL 1	MEAL 2	MEAL 3
☐ 4oz Lean Meat	☐ 4oz Lean Meat	☐ 4oz Lean Meat
☐ 3oz Starchy Veggie/Carbs	☐ 3oz Starchy Veggie/Carbs	☐ 3oz Starchy Veggie/Carbs
☐ **Unlimited** Non-Starchy Veggie	☐ **Unlimited** Non-Starchy Veggie	☐ **Unlimited** Non-Starchy Veggie
SNACK 1	SNACK 2	SNACK 3
☐ 12 - 30 Grams of Protein	☐ 12 - 30 Grams of Protein	☐ 12 - 30 Grams of Protein
☐ < 5 Grams of Fat	☐ < 5 Grams of Fat	☐ < 5 Grams of Fat

Dr. Melissa Ramsey DNP, MSN, RN, FNP-C

SUNDAY MEAL 1	MEAL 2	MEAL 3
☐ 4oz Lean Meat	☐ 4oz Lean Meat	☐ 4oz Lean Meat
☐ 3oz Starchy Veggie/Carbs	☐ 3oz Starchy Veggie/Carbs	☐ 3oz Starchy Veggie/Carbs
☐ **Unlimited** Non-Starchy Veggie	☐ **Unlimited** Non-Starchy Veggie	☐ **Unlimited** Non-Starchy Veggie
SNACK 1	SNACK 2	SNACK 3
☐ 12 - 30 Grams of Protein	☐ 12 - 30 Grams of Protein	☐ 12 - 30 Grams of Protein
☐ < 5 Grams of Fat	☐ < 5 Grams of Fat	☐ < 5 Grams of Fat

Male Meal Tracker

MONDAY MEAL 1	MEAL 2	MEAL 3
☐ 6oz Lean Meat	☐ 6oz Lean Meat	☐ 6oz Lean Meat
☐ 3oz Starchy Veggie/Carbs	☐ 3oz Starchy Veggie/Carbs	☐ 3oz Starchy Veggie/Carbs
☐ **Unlimited** Non-Starchy Veggie	☐ **Unlimited** Non-Starchy Veggie	☐ **Unlimited** Non-Starchy Veggie
SNACK 1	**SNACK 2**	**SNACK 3**
☐ 12 - 30 Grams of Protein	☐ 12 - 30 Grams of Protein	☐ 12 - 30 Grams of Protein
☐ < 5 Grams of Fat	☐ < 5 Grams of Fat	☐ < 5 Grams of Fat

TUESDAY MEAL 1	MEAL 2	MEAL 3
☐ 6oz Lean Meat	☐ 6oz Lean Meat	☐ 6oz Lean Meat
☐ 3oz Starchy Veggie/Carbs	☐ 3oz Starchy Veggie/Carbs	☐ 3oz Starchy Veggie/Carbs
☐ **Unlimited** Non-Starchy Veggie	☐ **Unlimited** Non-Starchy Veggie	☐ **Unlimited** Non-Starchy Veggie
SNACK 1	**SNACK 2**	**SNACK 3**
☐ 12 - 30 Grams of Protein	☐ 12 - 30 Grams of Protein	☐ 12 - 30 Grams of Protein
☐ < 5 Grams of Fat	☐ < 5 Grams of Fat	☐ < 5 Grams of Fat

WEDNESDAY MEAL 1	MEAL 2	MEAL 3
☐ 6oz Lean Meat ☐ 3oz Starchy Veggie/Carbs ☐ **Unlimited** Non-Starchy Veggie	☐ 6oz Lean Meat ☐ 3oz Starchy Veggie/Carbs ☐ **Unlimited** Non-Starchy Veggie	☐ 6oz Lean Meat ☐ 3oz Starchy Veggie/Carbs ☐ **Unlimited** Non-Starchy Veggie
SNACK 1	**SNACK 2**	**SNACK 3**
☐ 12 - 30 Grams of Protein ☐ < 5 Grams of Fat	☐ 12 - 30 Grams of Protein ☐ < 5 Grams of Fat	☐ 12 - 30 Grams of Protein ☐ < 5 Grams of Fat

THURSDAY MEAL 1	MEAL 2	MEAL 3
☐ 6oz Lean Meat ☐ 3oz Starchy Veggie/Carbs ☐ **Unlimited** Non-Starchy Veggie	☐ 6oz Lean Meat ☐ 3oz Starchy Veggie/Carbs ☐ **Unlimited** Non-Starchy Veggie	☐ 6oz Lean Meat ☐ 3oz Starchy Veggie/Carbs ☐ **Unlimited** Non-Starchy Veggie
SNACK 1	**SNACK 2**	**SNACK 3**
☐ 12 - 30 Grams of Protein ☐ < 5 Grams of Fat	☐ 12 - 30 Grams of Protein ☐ < 5 Grams of Fat	☐ 12 - 30 Grams of Protein ☐ < 5 Grams of Fat

FRIDAY MEAL 1	MEAL 2	MEAL 3
☐ 6oz Lean Meat	☐ 6oz Lean Meat	☐ 6oz Lean Meat
☐ 3oz Starchy Veggie/Carbs	☐ 3oz Starchy Veggie/Carbs	☐ 3oz Starchy Veggie/Carbs
☐ **Unlimited** Non-Starchy Veggie	☐ **Unlimited** Non-Starchy Veggie	☐ **Unlimited** Non-Starchy Veggie
SNACK 1	**SNACK 2**	**SNACK 3**
☐ 12 - 30 Grams of Protein	☐ 12 - 30 Grams of Protein	☐ 12 - 30 Grams of Protein
☐ < 5 Grams of Fat	☐ < 5 Grams of Fat	☐ < 5 Grams of Fat

SATURDAY MEAL 1	MEAL 2	MEAL 3
☐ 6oz Lean Meat	☐ 6oz Lean Meat	☐ 6oz Lean Meat
☐ 3oz Starchy Veggie/Carbs	☐ 3oz Starchy Veggie/Carbs	☐ 3oz Starchy Veggie/Carbs
☐ **Unlimited** Non-Starchy Veggie	☐ **Unlimited** Non-Starchy Veggie	☐ **Unlimited** Non-Starchy Veggie
SNACK 1	**SNACK 2**	**SNACK 3**
☐ 12 - 30 Grams of Protein	☐ 12 - 30 Grams of Protein	☐ 12 - 30 Grams of Protein
☐ < 5 Grams of Fat	☐ < 5 Grams of Fat	☐ < 5 Grams of Fat

SUNDAY MEAL 1	MEAL 2	MEAL 3
☐ 6oz Lean Meat	☐ 6oz Lean Meat	☐ 6oz Lean Meat
☐ 3oz Starchy Veggie/Carbs	☐ 3oz Starchy Veggie/Carbs	☐ 3oz Starchy Veggie/Carbs
☐ **Unlimited** Non-Starchy Veggie	☐ **Unlimited** Non-Starchy Veggie	☐ **Unlimited** Non-Starchy Veggie
SNACK 1	SNACK 2	SNACK 3
☐ 12 - 30 Grams of Protein	☐ 12 - 30 Grams of Protein	☐ 12 - 30 Grams of Protein
☐ < 5 Grams of Fat	☐ < 5 Grams of Fat	☐ < 5 Grams of Fat

The Habit Tracker

Habit:

	Sun	Mon	Tues	Wed	Thurs	Friday	Sat
Week 1							
Week 2							
Week 3							
Week 4							
Week 5							
Week 6							
Week 7							
Week 8							
Week 9							
Week 10							
Week 11							
Week 12							

<u>References</u>

Ammenheuser, M. (2023, December 20). Phantom fat: Body dysmorphic disorder after weight loss. My Vanderbilt Health. https://my.vanderbilthealth.com/phantom-fat-still-feel-oversized-even-losing-weight/

Andrew, R., Salunkhe, V., Yeap, S., & Wilson, A. (2020). Behavioral modification: Cognitive behavioral therapy in the management of obesity. Journal of Obesity & Eating Disorders, 6(2), 100–108. https://doi.org/10.21767/2471-8203.100079

Angelidi, A. M., Belanger, M. J., Lorinsky, M. K., & Mantzoros, C. S. (2021). The role of cognitive-behavioral therapy in weight management and obesity treatment: A systematic review. Metabolism, 120, 154800. https://doi.org/10.1016/j.metabol.2021.154800

Ansari, T., & Elhag, W. (2021). Factors contributing to obesity and weight management interventions. Journal of Family Medicine, 8(2), 56–63.

Ansari, T., Elhag, W., & Ahmed, R. (2020). Understanding obesity: Causes, management, and prevention. Public Health Research, 10(4), 145–152.

American Heart Association. (2018). Understanding childhood obesity: Facts and figures. https://www.heart.org

Avnieli Velfer, G., Kessler, A., & Shahar, D. R. (2019). Global trends in obesity prevalence: 2008–2016. Obesity Research & Clinical Practice, 13(3), 222–230.

Bahrami, Z., Heidari, A., & Cranney, J. (2022, September 28). Applying SMART goal intervention leads to greater goal attainment, need satisfaction and positive affect. Tech Science Press. https://doi.org/10.32604/ijmhp.2022.018954

Bray, G. A., Kim, K. K., Wilding, J. P., & World Obesity Federation. (2018). Obesity: A chronic relapsing progressive disease process: A position statement of the World Obesity Federation. Obesity Reviews, 18(7), 715–723. https://doi.org/10.1111/obr.12551

Campbell-Danesh, N. (2020). The psychology of weight loss: Cognitive behavioral strategies for success. British Journal of Health Psychology, 25(4), 1027–1045.

Chopra, S., Malhotra, A., & Ranjan, P. (2020). Behavioral interventions for weight loss: A systematic review of randomized controlled trials. Clinical Obesity, 10(3), e12362. https://doi.org/10.1111/cob.12362

Chopra, S., Ranjan, P., & Malhotra, A. (2021). Long-term efficacy of cognitive behavioral therapy for obesity management. Obesity Medicine, 22, 100317. https://doi.org/10.1016/j.obmed.2021.100317

Clear, J. (2018). Atomic habits: An easy & proven way to build good habits & break bad ones. Avery.

Dalle Grave, R., Calugi, S., & Marchesini, G. (2020). The role of cognitive-behavioral therapy in obesity management. International Journal of Obesity, 44, 1248–1257. https://doi.org/10.1038/s41366-020-0535-6

Dalle Grave, R., Calugi, S., Centis, E., El Ghoch, M., & Marchesini, G. (2015). Cognitive-behavioral strategies in the management of obesity. Neuropsychiatric Disease and Treatment, 11, 131–142. https://doi.org/10.2147/NDT.S81965

Everitt, H., Landau, S., O'Reilly, M., et al. (2022). Predictors of attrition in behavioral weight management programs. BMC Public Health, 22, 314. https://doi.org/10.1186/s12889-021-12493-5

Fernández-Álvarez, J., & Fernández-Álvarez, H. (2019). Cognitive behavioral therapy: Foundations and effectiveness. Frontiers in Psychology, 10, 2467. https://doi.org/10.3389/fpsyg.2019.02467

Gadde, K. M., & Atkins, D. (2020). Behavioral and pharmacologic treatments for obesity. The New England Journal of Medicine, 382(20), 1957–1968. https://doi.org/10.1056/NEJMra1910761

Grave, R. D., Calugi, S., & Marchesini, G. (2020). Behavioral therapy for obesity: New directions and future research. Frontiers in Endocrinology, 11, 571. https://doi.org/10.3389/fendo.2020.00571

Hall, K. D., & Kahan, S. (2018). Maintenance of lost weight and long-term management of obesity. Medical Clinics of North America, 102(1), 183–197. https://doi.org/10.1016/j.mcna.2017.08.012

Hall, K. D., & Kahan, S. (2019). Obesity prevention and treatment: Beyond the individual. Annals of the New York Academy of Sciences, 1461(1), 52–67. https://doi.org/10.1111/nyas.14142

Iłowiecka, K., Bąk, E., & Sidorowicz, M. (2021). CBT and weight reduction: Mechanisms and effects. International Journal of Environmental Research and Public Health, 18(21), 11465. https://doi.org/10.3390/ijerph182111465

Khanna, D., Gupta, R., & Sharma, R. (2022). Obesity: Definition, classification, and epidemiology. World Journal of Clinical Cases, 10(3), 641–652.

Krishnaswami, S., Beavers, K. M., & Lutes, L. D. (2018). Integrating CBT principles into obesity interventions. Journal of Behavioral Medicine, 41(2), 228–238. https://doi.org/10.1007/s10865-017-9898-5

LeBlanc, E. S., Patnode, C. D., Webber, E. M., Redmond, N., Rushkin, M., & O'Connor, E. A. (2018). Behavioral and pharmacotherapy weight loss interventions to prevent obesity-related morbidity and mortality in adults: Updated evidence report and systematic review for the US Preventive Services Task Force. JAMA, 320(11), 1172–1191. https://doi.org/10.1001/jama.2018.7777

Malik, V. S., Willett, W. C., & Hu, F. B. (2020). Global obesity: Trends, risk factors, and policy implications. Nature Reviews Endocrinology, 16, 239–248. https://doi.org/10.1038/s41574-019-0316-8

Mayle, A. (2021). Modern living and the obesity epidemic: Understanding lifestyle contributors. American Journal of Lifestyle Medicine, 15(6), 607–615.

Mayo Clinic. (2021). Childhood obesity. https://www.mayoclinic.org/diseases-conditions/childhood-obesity

Moraes, J. F. D., Gonçalves, M. S., & Santos, R. (2021). Effectiveness of cognitive behavioral therapy in obesity treatment: A meta-analysis. Psychology & Health, 36(8), 937–953. https://doi.org/10.1080/08870446.2020.1784350

Orvidas, K. (2019). How habits are formed: The psychology of routine behaviors. Psychology Today, 52(4), 22–29.

Pirotta, S., Joham, A. E., Moran, L. J., et al. (2019). Behavioral weight loss programs and attrition rates: Predictors and patterns. Obesity Research & Clinical Practice, 13(3), 223–231.

Ponzo, V., Pellegrini, M., & Bo, S. (2020). Habits, behavior, and obesity: The role of psychology. Nutrients, 12(10), 3038. https://doi.org/10.3390/nu12103038

Rand, C. S. (2017). The role of cognitive behavioral approaches in obesity treatment. Cognitive Therapy and Research, 41(5), 651–662. https://doi.org/10.1007/s10608-017-9852-4

Varkevisser, R. D. M., van Stralen, M. M., Kroeze, W., Ket, J. C. F., Steenhuis, I. H. M. (2019). Determinants of weight loss maintenance: A systematic review. Obesity Reviews, 20(2), 171–211. https://doi.org/10.1111/obr.12772

World Health Organization. (2020). Obesity and overweight. https://www.who.int/news-room/fact-sheets/detail/obesity-and-overweight

www.ingramcontent.com/pod-product-compliance
Lightning Source LLC
Chambersburg PA
CBHW032102020426
42335CB00011B/452